AYURVEDA FOR ENDOMORPHS

The Science of Self-Healing and How To Burn Fat And Boost Your Metabolism, To Achieve Holistic Health.

CELINA V. NEWTON

Copyright © 2024

All Rights Are Reserved

The content in this book may not be reproduced, duplicated, or transferred without the express written permission of the author or publisher. Under no circumstances will the publisher or author be held liable or legally responsible for any losses, expenditures, or damages incurred directly or indirectly as a consequence of the information included in this book.

Legal Remarks

Copyright protection applies to this publication. It is only intended for personal use. No piece of this work may be modified, distributed, sold, quoted, or paraphrased without the author's or publisher's consent.

Disclaimer Statement

Please keep in mind that the contents of this booklet are meant for educational and recreational purposes. Every effort has been made to offer accurate, up-to-date, reliable, and thorough information. There are, however, no stated or implied assurances of any kind. Readers understand that the author is providing competent counsel. The content in this book originates from several sources. Please seek the opinion of a Stop Storing Fat, Balance Hormones and Lose Weight Naturally by Eating More Food Through Delicious Recipes and just 7 days Meal Plan

competent professional before using any of the tactics outlined in this book. By reading this book, the reader agrees that the author will not be held accountable for any direct or indirect damages resulting from the use of the information contained therein, including, but not limited to, errors, omissions, or inaccuracies.

About the Author

CELINA V. NEWTON is a dedicated herbalist and holistic health expert, deeply passionate about using nature's bounty to promote healing and balance. Her journey into the world of natural medicine was inspired by the ancient wisdom of Ayurveda among other holistic traditions, leading her to explore the healing properties of plants and herbs extensively. Celina's approach to wellness is holistic, considering the emotional, mental, and spiritual facets of health alongside the physical.

With a background in botany and holistic medicine, Celina crafts personalized herbal treatments that cater to the individual needs of her clients, aiming to restore harmony and wellness from within. She is known for her compassionate approach, taking the time to truly understand each person's unique situation and wellness goals.

CELINA V. NEWTON is also a fervent advocate for education in herbal and holistic health practices. She conducts workshops and seminars, sharing her knowledge on how to incorporate natural remedies and mindful practices into everyday life, promoting a healthier, more sustainable way of living.

As an author, Celina's work breaks down the complexities of herbal medicine and holistic therapies, making them accessible to all. Her writing encourages people to embrace natural remedies and holistic health practices, empowering them to take charge of their well-being.

Personal experience with the healing power of herbs and holistic practices has fueled Celina's dedication. Her work is not just her profession; it's her passion and life's mission, making her a trusted figure in the natural health community. She continues to inspire those seeking a harmonious, balanced approach to health and wellness.

TABLE OF CONTENTS

Introduction 5
Chapter 1 8
   Understanding Ayurveda 8
   Overview of Endomorph Body Type 11
Chapter 2 14
Ayurvedic Principles for Weight Management 14
   Balancing Doshas (Vata, Pitta, Kapha) 14
   Importance of Agni (Digestive Fire) 16
Chapter 3 19
Identifying Your Dominant Dosha 19
   Dosha Assessment for Endomorphs 19
   Personalizing Ayurvedic Recommendations 21
Chapter 4 24
Ayurvedic Diet for Endomorphs 24
   Ayurvedic Breakfast Recipes for Endomorphs 24
   Ayurvedic Lunch Recipes for Endomorphs 39
   Ayurvedic Dinner Recipes for Endomorphs 54
   Ayurvedic Dessert Recipes for Endomorphs 79
Chapter 5 92
Sample Meal Plan 92
Chapter 6 102
Herbal Remedies for Weight Management 102
   Ayurvedic Herbs for Metabolism and Digestion 102
   Herbal Formulas for Endomorphs 105
Conclusion 109

INTRODUCTION

Life is full of unseen battles, and among these is the personal struggle of being an endomorph, a challenge that goes far beyond the surface. This story is about Nelly, who stands for many facing daily confrontations with their weight and self-perception. Her journey isn't merely about losing weight; it's a deeper quest for self-esteem and recognizing her inherent beauty.

Nelly's early years were filled with the usual joys, aspirations, and a boundless zest for life. However, as she transitioned into her teenage years, she noticed her body evolving differently from her friends. While they remained naturally slim, Nelly battled against gaining extra weight, turning shopping trips and social events into stressful episodes filled with self-comparison and increasing insecurity.

With time, these struggles only intensified. Nelly tried every new diet, from strict calorie counting to cutting out entire food categories, yet the weight persistently returned, eroding her confidence and leaving her feeling defeated by her own reflection. This cycle of effort and disappointment led Nelly to brace herself for a life of ongoing dissatisfaction, watching as her dreams of vibrancy and self-assurance were overshadowed by doubt and gloom.

Yet, in her darkest moments, Nelly discovered a sliver of hope in Ayurveda, an ancient system promising holistic healing. This discovery was not just a turning point; it was a lifeline, offering her the understanding and solutions that had eluded her for so long.

Ayurveda brought Nelly much more than a weight loss regimen; it provided a journey towards self-discovery and empowerment. Through its principles, Nelly learned to honor her unique body type, transforming her endomorphic characteristics from a source of embarrassment to one of strength.

Immersing herself in Ayurvedic wisdom, Nelly uncovered a wealth of knowledge that reshaped her approach to health and well-being. She began nourishing her body with foods that supported her from within, shifting from a mindset of deprivation to one of abundance.

But Ayurveda offered Nelly more than dietary guidance; it presented a holistic way of living. She integrated ancient rituals and practices into her daily routine, aligning with the natural rhythms of her body and the environment around her.

Gradually, Nelly experienced a transformation. She felt lighter, not just in body but in spirit, and the mirror reflected a woman radiating inner strength and beauty.

Nelly's path was not without its hurdles, facing days filled with doubt and old, negative voices trying to pull her back. Nonetheless, she stood unwavering, fortified by the profound insights and resilience she had cultivated.

Today, Nelly exemplifies the healing and transformative potential of Ayurveda. Her journey continues with renewed purpose and hope, a testament to the belief that the most significant journey is the one that leads inward.

Let Nelly's story be a source of inspiration. No matter the darkness, transformation awaits those willing to embrace change. With an open heart and courage, embark on your path, for within you lies the potential for a life of vitality, joy, and fulfillment.

CHAPTER 1

Understanding Ayurveda

Ayurveda, often referred to as the "science of life" or the "knowledge of longevity," is an ancient holistic healing system that originated in India over 5,000 years ago. Rooted in the belief that health is a harmonious balance between body, mind, and spirit, Ayurveda offers a comprehensive approach to well-being that encompasses diet, lifestyle, herbal remedies, and therapeutic practices.

At the heart of Ayurveda lies the principle of the five elements—earth, water, fire, air, and ether—each representing different qualities and energies within the body. According to Ayurvedic philosophy, the human body is composed of these elements in varying proportions, giving rise to three primary constitutional types known as doshas: Vata, Pitta, and Kapha.

Vata dosha is associated with the elements of air and ether and governs movement, creativity, and communication. Pitta dosha, representing fire and water, governs metabolism, digestion, and transformation. Kapha dosha, composed of earth and water, governs structure, stability, and nourishment.

Understanding one's unique doshic constitution is fundamental to Ayurvedic practice. By identifying the dominant doshas within an individual, Ayurveda provides personalized guidelines for maintaining health and preventing disease. Each person's constitution is as unique as their fingerprint, and Ayurveda recognizes that what works for one individual may not necessarily work for another.

Ayurveda emphasizes the interconnectedness of all aspects of life, recognizing that physical health is inseparable from mental, emotional, and spiritual well-being. The ancient texts of Ayurveda describe the importance of cultivating balance in all areas of life, from diet and exercise to relationships and spiritual practices.

Central to Ayurvedic philosophy is the concept of prakriti, or one's inherent nature, which is determined by the doshic constitution present at birth. Prakriti influences an individual's physical characteristics, temperament, and susceptibility to disease. Understanding one's prakriti allows for a deeper insight into one's unique needs and vulnerabilities, guiding personalized approaches to health and healing.

Ayurveda offers a wealth of holistic remedies for maintaining health and addressing imbalances. Herbal medicine plays a central role in Ayurvedic treatment, with thousands of plant-based remedies used to support digestion, boost immunity, and promote vitality. Ayurvedic herbs such as turmeric, ashwagandha, and triphala have gained popularity worldwide for their potent healing properties.

In addition to herbal medicine, Ayurveda encompasses a wide range of therapeutic modalities, including massage, yoga, meditation, and detoxification practices. Ayurvedic massage, known as abhyanga, is performed using warm oils infused with medicinal herbs to nourish the skin, soothe the nervous system, and promote relaxation. Yoga and meditation are integral components of Ayurvedic practice, helping to balance the doshas, calm the mind, and cultivate inner peace.

Ayurveda recognizes the importance of seasonal rhythms and cycles in maintaining health and harmony. Each season is associated with unique qualities and influences that can impact the doshas. By aligning with the rhythms of nature, Ayurveda offers guidance for adapting diet, lifestyle, and self-care practices to support optimal health throughout the year.

In summary, Ayurveda offers a profound understanding of health and healing that transcends conventional medicine.

Rooted in ancient wisdom and timeless principles, Ayurveda provides a holistic framework for promoting well-being and preventing disease. By embracing the principles of Ayurveda, individuals can cultivate balance, vitality, and harmony in all aspects of life.

Overview of Endomorph Body Type

The concept of somatotypes, or body types, has been widely studied and discussed in the field of anthropology and psychology. Introduced by American psychologist William Sheldon in the 1940s, somatotypes categorize individuals into three primary body types: endomorph, mesomorph, and ectomorph.

Endomorphs are characterized by a softer, rounder physique with a tendency to store excess body fat. They typically have a larger bone structure, wider hips, and a higher percentage of body fat compared to mesomorphs and ectomorphs. Endomorphs often struggle with weight management and may find it challenging to lose fat and build lean muscle mass.

From a physiological standpoint, endomorphs tend to have a slower metabolism and may be more prone to insulin resistance and hormonal imbalances. These factors can contribute to difficulties in maintaining a healthy weight and may increase the risk of obesity-related health conditions such as diabetes, heart disease, and metabolic syndrome.

Psychologically, endomorphs may experience challenges related to body image and self-esteem. Society's idealized standards of beauty often prioritize slimness and muscularity, leaving endomorphs feeling marginalized and misunderstood. The pervasive influence of media and advertising perpetuates unrealistic body ideals, further exacerbating feelings of inadequacy and shame.

Despite the challenges they face, endomorphs possess unique strengths and qualities that deserve recognition and celebration. Endomorphs are often described as warm, nurturing, and empathetic individuals with a strong capacity for emotional connection. Their generous nature and compassionate spirit enrich the lives of those around them, fostering deep bonds of friendship and community.

Understanding one's somatotype, including the characteristics and challenges associated with being an endomorph, is an important step towards achieving greater self-awareness and acceptance. Rather than viewing their body type as a limitation, endomorphs can embrace their unique attributes and work towards cultivating a positive body image and sense of self-worth.

In the journey towards health and well-being, endomorphs can benefit from adopting a holistic approach that addresses both physical and emotional aspects of wellness. By focusing on nourishing whole foods, engaging in regular physical activity, managing stress, and prioritizing self-care, endomorphs can support their body's natural healing mechanisms and promote vitality from within.

It's important to recognize that there is no one-size-fits-all approach to health and fitness. Each individual is unique, and what works for one person may not necessarily work for another. By honoring their body's innate wisdom and embracing their inherent worth, endomorphs can reclaim ownership of their health and embark on a journey of self-discovery and empowerment.

CHAPTER 2

AYURVEDIC PRINCIPLES FOR WEIGHT MANAGEMENT

Ayurveda, the ancient healing system originating from India, offers a profound understanding of weight management that extends beyond calorie counting and restrictive diets. Rooted in the principle of holistic health, Ayurveda recognizes that maintaining a healthy weight is not just about physical appearance but is essential for overall well-being. Ayurvedic principles for weight management focus on restoring balance to the body, mind, and spirit, addressing the underlying imbalances that contribute to weight gain.

Balancing Doshas (Vata, Pitta, Kapha)

Central to Ayurvedic principles for weight management is the concept of doshas—Vata, Pitta, and Kapha—which represent different combinations of the five elements (earth, water, fire, air, and ether) present in the human body. Each dosha governs specific physiological functions and qualities, and an imbalance in any of the doshas can lead to weight-related issues.

Vata dosha, associated with the elements of air and ether, governs movement, communication, and creativity. When

Vata is out of balance, individuals may experience irregular digestion, anxiety, and difficulty gaining weight. Pitta dosha, representing fire and water, governs metabolism, digestion, and transformation. Imbalances in Pitta can manifest as excessive hunger, inflammation, and metabolic disorders. Kapha dosha, composed of earth and water, governs structure, stability, and nourishment. When Kapha is imbalanced, individuals may experience sluggish digestion, weight gain, and lethargy.

Balancing the doshas is essential for promoting healthy weight management in Ayurveda. This involves identifying the predominant doshas in an individual and implementing lifestyle, dietary, and herbal remedies to restore balance. For example, individuals with excess Vata may benefit from incorporating grounding foods such as root vegetables, warm soups, and cooked grains into their diet. Pitta-predominant individuals may benefit from cooling foods such as leafy greens, cucumbers, and coconut water to pacify excess heat in the body. Kapha-dominant individuals may benefit from light, dry foods such as legumes, bitter greens, and spicy herbs to stimulate digestion and reduce heaviness.

Importance of Agni (Digestive Fire)

In Ayurveda, Agni—often referred to as the digestive fire—is considered the cornerstone of health and vitality. Responsible for the digestion, absorption, and assimilation of nutrients, Agni plays a crucial role in determining overall metabolic efficiency and weight management.

Agni is influenced by the quality of food consumed, the strength of the digestive organs, and the individual's doshic constitution. When Agni is strong and balanced, food is digested efficiently, toxins are eliminated effectively, and energy levels remain stable throughout the day. However, when Agni is weak or imbalanced, digestive disturbances, nutrient deficiencies, and weight gain can occur.

Ayurveda recognizes several factors that can impair Agni and disrupt digestive function, including poor dietary choices, irregular eating habits, stress, and environmental toxins. Processed foods, refined sugars, excessive fats, and heavy, hard-to-digest foods can overwhelm Agni and lead to the accumulation of toxins (ama) in the body, hindering metabolic function and contributing to weight gain.

To support healthy Agni and promote optimal digestion, Ayurveda offers dietary guidelines and lifestyle practices that nourish and strengthen the digestive fire. Choosing whole, unprocessed foods that are fresh, seasonal, and locally sourced helps provide essential nutrients and support digestive function. Eating mindfully, in a calm and relaxed environment, allows the body to fully engage its digestive processes and optimize nutrient absorption.

In addition to dietary considerations, Ayurveda recommends incorporating herbs and spices that enhance Agni and promote digestive health. Digestive stimulants such as ginger, black pepper, cumin, and cardamom can help kindle the digestive fire, improve appetite, and alleviate digestive discomfort. Herbal formulations such as triphala—a combination of three fruits known for their cleansing and rejuvenating properties—support regular bowel movements and help remove toxins from the body.

Ayurveda also emphasizes the importance of maintaining a balanced lifestyle that supports Agni and promotes overall well-being. Establishing regular meal times, prioritizing adequate hydration, and incorporating stress management techniques such as meditation, yoga, and deep breathing exercises can help maintain healthy digestive function and support weight management efforts.

By cultivating awareness of Agni and making conscious choices that support optimal digestion, individuals can unlock the key to vibrant health, vitality, and sustainable weight management. Ayurveda offers a holistic approach to wellness that honors the interconnectedness of body, mind, and spirit, providing a pathway to lifelong health and vitality.

CHAPTER 3

IDENTIFYING YOUR DOMINANT DOSHA

Understanding your dominant dosha is a fundamental aspect of Ayurvedic practice. The doshas—Vata, Pitta, and Kapha—represent the fundamental energies that govern all biological functions within the body. Each person is born with a unique combination of these doshas, which influences their physical, mental, and emotional characteristics.

Dosha Assessment for Endomorphs

Endomorphs, characterized by a tendency to store excess body fat and a slower metabolism, often have specific patterns and imbalances within their doshic constitution. While everyone possesses all three doshas to varying degrees, endomorphs may find that certain doshas are more prominent or imbalanced in their physiology.

To assess your doshic constitution as an endomorph, consider the following factors:

1. **Physical Characteristics**: Endomorphs typically have a larger frame, softer features, and a tendency to gain weight easily. They may have a rounded body shape,

with wider hips and shoulders and a propensity to store fat around the abdomen, thighs, and buttocks.

2. **Metabolic Patterns**: Endomorphs often have a slower metabolism, which can contribute to difficulties in losing weight and maintaining a healthy body composition. They may experience challenges with digestion and assimilation, leading to sluggishness and lethargy.

3. **Emotional Traits**: Endomorphs may exhibit characteristics associated with Kapha dosha, such as calmness, patience, and emotional stability. However, they may also struggle with tendencies towards lethargy, attachment, and resistance to change.

4. **Psychological Tendencies**: Endomorphs may be prone to emotional eating, seeking comfort and solace in food during times of stress or emotional upheaval. They may also experience feelings of heaviness, stagnation, and inertia, both physically and mentally.

5. **Health Patterns**: Endomorphs may be more susceptible to conditions associated with Kapha dosha, such as obesity, diabetes, high cholesterol, and respiratory disorders. They may also experience challenges related to hormonal imbalances, insulin resistance, and metabolic syndrome.

By assessing these factors and recognizing the predominant doshic influences within your body and mind, you can gain insight into your unique constitution as an endomorph and identify areas of imbalance that may require attention and support.

Personalizing Ayurvedic Recommendations

Once you have identified your dominant dosha as an endomorph, you can begin to personalize your Ayurvedic recommendations to support balance and well-being. Ayurveda offers a wealth of holistic practices and remedies tailored to individual doshic constitutions, helping to restore harmony and vitality to body, mind, and spirit.

Here are some personalized Ayurvedic recommendations for endomorphs:

1. **Diet and Nutrition**: As an endomorph, focus on a diet that is nourishing, balanced, and supportive of your unique constitution. Emphasize whole, unprocessed foods that are light, warm, and easy to digest. Favor cooked vegetables, grains, lean proteins, and healthy fats, while minimizing heavy, oily, and sweet foods that can exacerbate Kapha imbalances.

2. **Digestive Support**: Support healthy digestion and metabolism by incorporating digestive spices and herbs

into your meals, such as ginger, cumin, coriander, and fenugreek. Consider drinking warm water with lemon first thing in the morning to stimulate digestion and detoxification.

3. **Lifestyle Practices**: Establish a daily routine that promotes balance and vitality. Wake up early, engage in regular exercise, and prioritize activities that uplift and energize you. Incorporate yoga, meditation, and deep breathing exercises to calm the mind, reduce stress, and enhance overall well-being.

4. **Herbal Remedies**: Explore Ayurvedic herbs and supplements that support weight management, metabolism, and hormonal balance. Herbs such as triphala, guggul, and guduchi may be beneficial for promoting detoxification, boosting metabolism, and supporting healthy weight loss.

5. **Detoxification**: Consider incorporating periodic detoxification practices to remove accumulated toxins and stagnation from the body. Ayurvedic detox techniques such as fasting, herbal cleanses, and oil pulling can help to rejuvenate the digestive system, improve energy levels, and promote clarity of mind.

6. **Mind-Body Practices**: Cultivate mindfulness and self-awareness through practices such as meditation, journaling, and visualization. Develop a positive mindset, cultivate self-compassion, and practice gratitude for the blessings in your life.

7. **Self-Care Rituals**: Prioritize self-care and nurturing activities that replenish your energy and nourish your soul. Take time for relaxation, massage, and aromatherapy to soothe the senses and promote deep restorative rest.

CHAPTER 4

AYURVEDIC DIET FOR ENDOMORPHS

Ayurvedic Breakfast Recipes for Endomorphs

1. Quinoa Porridge with Warm Spices

Ingredients:

- 1 cup quinoa
- 2 cups almond milk
- 1 teaspoon cinnamon
- ½ teaspoon cardamom
- 1 tablespoon honey
- Fresh berries for garnish

Preparation Time: 5 minutes
Cooking Time: 15 minutes
Serving Time: 20 minutes

Instructions:

1. Rinse quinoa and cook in almond milk with spices until tender.
2. Sweeten with honey and top with fresh berries.

Nutritional Information:

- Protein: 10g
- Fiber: 5g
- Calories: 300

Serving Suggestions:

- Add sliced almonds for crunch.
- Sprinkle with chia seeds for added nutrition.

2. Ayurvedic Vegetable Omelette

Ingredients:

- 3 eggs
- ¼ cup chopped bell peppers
- ¼ cup chopped spinach
- ¼ teaspoon turmeric
- Salt and pepper to taste
- Fresh herbs for garnish

Preparation Time: 10 minutes
Cooking Time: 5 minutes
Serving Time: 15 minutes

Instructions:

1. Whisk eggs and mix in vegetables and spices.
2. Cook in a non-stick pan until set. Garnish with fresh herbs.

Nutritional Information:

- Protein: 15g
- Fiber: 3g
- Calories: 220

Serving Suggestions:

- Serve with a side of sliced avocado.
- Pair with whole grain toast.

3. Chia Seed Pudding with Almond Butter

Ingredients:

- 3 tablespoons chia seeds
- 1 cup almond milk
- 1 tablespoon almond butter
- ½ teaspoon vanilla extract
- Sliced bananas for topping

Preparation Time: 5 minutes (plus chilling time)
Cooking Time: 0 minutes
Serving Time: 5 minutes (after chilling)

Instructions:

1. Mix chia seeds, almond milk, almond butter, and vanilla. Refrigerate overnight.
2. Top with sliced bananas before serving.

Nutritional Information:

- Protein: 8g
- Fiber: 12g
- Calories: 250

Serving Suggestions:

- Sprinkle with crushed nuts for added texture.
- Drizzle with honey for sweetness.

4. Sweet Potato and Kale Breakfast Bowl

Ingredients:

- 1 cup roasted sweet potatoes
- 1 cup sautéed kale
- 2 poached eggs
- ¼ teaspoon cumin
- Salt and pepper to taste

Preparation Time: 15 minutes
Cooking Time: 20 minutes
Serving Time: 35 minutes

Instructions:

1. Roast sweet potatoes and sauté kale in olive oil with cumin.
2. Poach eggs and serve over the vegetables.

Nutritional Information:

- Protein: 14g
- Fiber: 6g
- Calories: 280

Serving Suggestions:
- Drizzle with a tahini dressing.
- Top with a sprinkle of nutritional yeast.

5. Millet Pancakes with Berry Compote

Ingredients:
- 1 cup millet flour
- ½ cup almond milk
- 1 tablespoon coconut oil
- ½ cup mixed berries (for compote)
- 1 tablespoon maple syrup

Preparation Time: 10 minutes
Cooking Time: 15 minutes
Serving Time: 25 minutes

Instructions:
1. Mix millet flour, almond milk, and coconut oil to make the pancake batter.
2. Cook pancakes and top with mixed berry compote and maple syrup.

Nutritional Information:
- Protein: 7g
- Fiber: 4g
- Calories: 220

Serving Suggestions:

- Serve with a dollop of Greek yogurt.
- Sprinkle with crushed pistachios.

6. Turmeric Ginger Smoothie Bowl

Ingredients:

- 1 frozen banana
- ½ cup frozen mango chunks
- ½ cup almond milk
- 1 teaspoon turmeric powder
- 1 teaspoon grated ginger
- Toppings: sliced kiwi, shredded coconut

Preparation Time: 5 minutes
Cooking Time: 0 minutes
Serving Time: 5 minutes

Instructions:

1. Blend frozen banana, mango chunks, almond milk, turmeric, and ginger until smooth.
2. Pour into a bowl and top with sliced kiwi and shredded coconut.

Nutritional Information:

- Protein: 5g
- Fiber: 6g
- Calories: 230

Serving Suggestions:

- Add a sprinkle of granola for crunch.
- Drizzle with honey or agave syrup for added sweetness.

7. Warm Apple Cinnamon Oats

Ingredients:

- ½ cup rolled oats
- 1 cup water or almond milk
- ½ apple, diced
- ½ teaspoon cinnamon
- 1 tablespoon honey or maple syrup

Preparation Time: 5 minutes
Cooking Time: 10 minutes
Serving Time: 15 minutes

Instructions:

1. Cook rolled oats with water or almond milk until creamy.
2. Stir in diced apple, cinnamon, and sweetener of choice until heated through.

Nutritional Information:

- Protein: 6g
- Fiber: 4g
- Calories: 220

Serving Suggestions:

- Top with a spoonful of almond butter.
- Garnish with a sprinkle of chopped nuts.

8. Spinach and Mushroom Breakfast Wrap

Ingredients:

- 2 whole grain tortillas
- 1 cup sautéed spinach
- ½ cup sautéed mushrooms
- 2 eggs, scrambled
- ¼ cup shredded cheese (optional)

Preparation Time: 10 minutes
Cooking Time: 10 minutes
Serving Time: 20 minutes

Instructions:

1. Fill tortillas with sautéed spinach, mushrooms, scrambled eggs, and shredded cheese (if using).
2. Roll up and serve warm.

Nutritional Information:

- Protein: 12g
- Fiber: 4g
- Calories: 300

Serving Suggestions:

- Serve with a side of salsa or avocado slices.
- Wrap in parchment paper for an on-the-go breakfast option.

9. Coconut Chia Seed Pudding

Ingredients:

- 3 tablespoons chia seeds
- 1 cup coconut milk
- 1 tablespoon maple syrup
- ½ teaspoon vanilla extract
- Sliced mango for topping

Preparation Time: 5 minutes (plus chilling time)
Cooking Time: 0 minutes
Serving Time: 5 minutes (after chilling)

Instructions:

1. Mix chia seeds, coconut milk, maple syrup, and vanilla. Refrigerate until thickened.
2. Top with sliced mango before serving.

Nutritional Information:

- Protein: 6g
- Fiber: 8g
- Calories: 240

Serving Suggestions:

- Garnish with toasted coconut flakes.
- Add a sprinkle of ground cinnamon for flavour.

10. Ayurvedic Breakfast Salad

Ingredients:

- 2 cups mixed greens
- ½ cup cooked quinoa
- ¼ cup chickpeas, drained and rinsed
- ¼ cup diced cucumber
- ¼ cup cherry tomatoes, halved
- Dressing: olive oil, lemon juice, salt, and pepper

Preparation Time: 10 minutes
Cooking Time: 15 minutes (for quinoa)
Serving Time: 25 minutes

Instructions:

1. Toss mixed greens, cooked quinoa, chickpeas, cucumber, and cherry tomatoes in a bowl.
2. Drizzle with olive oil, lemon juice, salt, and pepper for dressing.

Nutritional Information:

- Protein: 8g
- Fiber: 6g
- Calories: 280

Serving Suggestions:

- Top with sliced avocado or boiled egg.
- Sprinkle with fresh herbs like cilantro or parsley.

11. Almond Butter Banana Toast

Ingredients:

- 2 slices whole grain bread
- 2 tablespoons almond butter
- 1 banana, sliced
- Drizzle of honey

Preparation Time: 5 minutes
Cooking Time: 0 minutes
Serving Time: 5 minutes

Instructions:

1. Toast whole grain bread until golden brown.
2. Spread almond butter on toast and top with sliced banana. Drizzle with honey.

Nutritional Information:

- Protein: 7g
- Fiber: 5g
- Calories: 250

Serving Suggestions:

- Sprinkle with cinnamon for added flavour.
- Serve with a glass of almond milk or herbal tea.

12. Ayurvedic Tofu Scramble

Ingredients:

- ½ block firm tofu, crumbled
- ¼ cup diced bell peppers
- ¼ cup diced onions
- ¼ teaspoon turmeric
- Salt and pepper to taste
- Fresh parsley for garnish

Preparation Time: 10 minutes
Cooking Time: 10 minutes
Serving Time: 20 minutes

Instructions:

1. Sauté diced bell peppers and onions until softened.
2. Add crumbled tofu, turmeric, salt, and pepper. Cook until heated through.
3. Garnish with fresh parsley before serving.

Nutritional Information:

- Protein: 15g
- Fiber: 4g
- Calories: 280

Serving Suggestions:

- Serve with whole grain toast or tortillas.
- Add sliced avocado for creaminess.

13. Berry and Yogurt Parfait

Ingredients:

- ½ cup Greek yogurt
- ¼ cup granola
- ¼ cup mixed berries (strawberries, blueberries, raspberries)
- Drizzle of honey or maple syrup

Preparation Time: 5 minutes
Cooking Time: 0 minutes
Serving Time: 5 minutes

Instructions:

1. Layer Greek yogurt, granola, and mixed berries in a glass or bowl.
2. Drizzle with honey or maple syrup before serving.

Nutritional Information:

- Protein: 12g
- Fiber: 4g
- Calories: 270

Serving Suggestions:

- Top with a sprinkle of chia seeds for added nutrition.
- Garnish with fresh mint leaves for freshness.

14. Ayurvedic Turmeric Latte

Ingredients:

- 1 cup almond milk
- 1 teaspoon turmeric powder
- ½ teaspoon cinnamon
- Pinch of black pepper
- 1 teaspoon honey or maple syrup

Preparation Time: 5 minutes
Cooking Time: 5 minutes
Serving Time: 10 minutes

Instructions:

1. Heat almond milk in a saucepan with turmeric, cinnamon, and black pepper.
2. Sweeten with honey or maple syrup. Stir well and serve hot.

Nutritional Information:

- Protein: 3g
- Fiber: 1g
- Calories: 100

Serving Suggestions:

- Sprinkle with a dash of nutmeg for added flavour.
- Serve with a cinnamon stick for stirring.

15. Ayurvedic Avocado Toast

Ingredients:

- 2 slices whole grain bread
- 1 ripe avocado, mashed
- Squeeze of lemon juice
- Sprinkle of red pepper flakes
- Salt and pepper to taste

Preparation Time: 5 minutes
Cooking Time: 0 minutes
Serving Time: 5 minutes

Instructions:

1. Toast whole grain bread until golden brown.
2. Spread mashed avocado on toast and season with lemon juice, red pepper flakes, salt, and pepper.

Nutritional Information:

- Protein: 6g
- Fiber: 8g
- Calories: 280

Serving Suggestions:

- Top with sliced cherry tomatoes for freshness.
- Garnish with microgreens or sprouts for added nutrients.

Ayurvedic Lunch Recipes for Endomorphs

1. Quinoa and Vegetable Bowl

Ingredients:

- 1 cup quinoa
- Mixed vegetables (bell peppers, zucchini, carrots)
- 1 tablespoon ghee
- Cumin seeds, coriander powder, turmeric
- Salt and pepper to taste

Preparation Time: 10 minutes
Cooking Time: 20 minutes
Serving Time: Lunch

Instructions:

1. Rinse quinoa and cook according to package instructions.
2. In a pan, sauté mixed vegetables in ghee with cumin seeds, coriander powder, turmeric, salt, and pepper.
3. Combine cooked quinoa and vegetables. Serve warm.

Nutritional Information:

- High in protein, fibre, and essential nutrients.

Serving Suggestions:

- Top with fresh cilantro and a squeeze of lemon.
- Add a side of cucumber raita for a cooling element.

2. Spiced Lentil Soup

Ingredients:

- 1 cup red lentils
- Onion, tomatoes, garlic, ginger
- Garam masala, cumin, coriander
- Vegetable broth
- Fresh cilantro for garnish

Preparation Time: 15 minutes
Cooking Time: 30 minutes
Serving Time: Lunch

Instructions:

1. Sauté onions, garlic, and ginger. Add tomatoes and spices.
2. Add red lentils and vegetable broth. Simmer until lentils are cooked.
3. Garnish with fresh cilantro before serving.

Nutritional Information:

- Rich in protein, fibre, and iron.

Serving Suggestions:

- Serve with brown rice for a complete meal.
- Drizzle with a spoonful of plain yogurt.

3. Stir-Fried Tofu with Veggies

Ingredients:

- Firm tofu, cubed
- Mixed vegetables (broccoli, bell peppers, snap peas)
- Tamari sauce, sesame oil, ginger
- Brown rice or quinoa

Preparation Time: 15 minutes
Cooking Time: 20 minutes
Serving Time: Lunch

Instructions:

1. Press tofu to remove excess water, then stir-fry with tamari, sesame oil, and ginger.
2. Add mixed vegetables and continue stir-frying until cooked.
3. Serve over brown rice or quinoa.

Nutritional Information:

- Excellent source of plant-based protein and antioxidants.

Serving Suggestions:

- Garnish with sesame seeds and green onions.
- Drizzle with a tahini-based sauce for added flavour.

4. Chickpea and Spinach Curry

Ingredients:

- Canned chickpeas
- Spinach, tomatoes, onions
- Curry spices (turmeric, cumin, coriander)
- Coconut milk
- Basmati rice

Preparation Time: 15 minutes
Cooking Time: 25 minutes
Serving Time: Lunch

Instructions:

1. Sauté onions, add spices, then stir in tomatoes.
2. Add chickpeas, spinach, and coconut milk. Simmer until spinach wilts.
3. Serve over basmati rice.

Nutritional Information:

- Rich in fibre, plant-based protein, and iron.

Serving Suggestions:

- Sprinkle with fresh chopped cilantro.
- Serve with a side of mango chutney for sweetness.

5. Roasted Sweet Potato and Lentil Salad

Ingredients:

- Sweet potatoes, cubed
- Green lentils, cooked
- Cherry tomatoes, cucumber, red onion
- Olive oil, lemon juice, Dijon mustard

Preparation Time: 20 minutes
Cooking Time: 30 minutes
Serving Time: Lunch

Instructions:

1. Roast sweet potatoes until tender.
2. Mix with cooked green lentils, cherry tomatoes, cucumber, and red onion.
3. Toss with olive oil, lemon juice, and Dijon mustard dressing.

Nutritional Information:

- Packed with fibre, vitamins, and antioxidants.

Serving Suggestions:

1. Top with crumbled feta or goat cheese.
2. Serve on a bed of mixed greens for added freshness.

6. Mung Bean Stew

Ingredients:

- Mung beans, soaked
- Carrots, celery, tomatoes
- Turmeric, cumin, ginger
- Vegetable broth
- Fresh parsley for garnish

Preparation Time: 15 minutes
Cooking Time: 40 minutes
Serving Time: Lunch

Instructions:

1. Sauté carrots, celery, and tomatoes. Add spices.
2. Add soaked mung beans and vegetable broth. Simmer until beans are tender.
3. Garnish with fresh parsley before serving.

Nutritional Information:

- High in protein, fibre, and essential nutrients.

Serving Suggestions:

- Serve with a dollop of plain Greek yogurt.
- Sprinkle with a dash of lemon juice for brightness.

7. Sesame Ginger Brown Rice with Vegetables

Ingredients:

- Brown rice, cooked
- Mixed vegetables (Bok choy, carrots, snow peas)
- Sesame oil, soy sauce, ginger
- Sesame seeds for garnish

Preparation Time: 15 minutes
Cooking Time: 20 minutes
Serving Time: Lunch

Instructions:

1. Sauté mixed vegetables in sesame oil and ginger.
2. Add cooked brown rice and soy sauce. Stir until well combined.
3. Garnish with sesame seeds before serving.

Nutritional Information:

- Provides fibre, antioxidants, and essential minerals.

Serving Suggestions:

- Add a dash of Sriracha for a spicy kick.
- Serve with a side of pickled ginger for added flavour.

8. Cauliflower and Chickpea Masala

Ingredients:

- Cauliflower florets
- Chickpeas, cooked
- Onion, garlic, tomatoes
- Garam masala, turmeric, cumin
- Coconut milk

Preparation Time: 20 minutes
Cooking Time: 30 minutes
Serving Time: Lunch

Instructions:

1. Sauté onions, garlic, and tomatoes. Add spices.
2. Add cauliflower florets and cooked chickpeas.
3. Stir in coconut milk and simmer until cauliflower is tender.

Nutritional Information:

- Rich in fibre, plant-based protein, and anti-inflammatory spices.

Serving Suggestions:

- Garnish with fresh cilantro and a squeeze of lime.
- Serve over quinoa or brown rice for a complete meal.

9. Turmeric-Ginger Lentil Soup

Ingredients:

- Red lentils
- Carrots, celery, onion
- Turmeric, ginger, cumin
- Vegetable broth
- Coconut milk

Preparation Time: 15 minutes
Cooking Time: 25 minutes
Serving Time: Lunch

Instructions:

1. Sauté carrots, celery, and onion. Add spices.
2. Add red lentils and vegetable broth. Simmer until lentils are cooked.
3. Stir in coconut milk before serving.

Nutritional Information:

- Provides protein, fibre, and anti-inflammatory properties.

Serving Suggestions:

- Serve with a dollop of Greek yogurt.
- Garnish with fresh parsley or cilantro.

10. Ayurvedic Chickpea Salad

Ingredients:

- Canned chickpeas
- Cucumber, tomatoes, red onion
- Lemon juice, olive oil, cumin
- Fresh mint or parsley for garnish

Preparation Time: 15 minutes
Cooking Time: 0 minutes
Serving Time: Lunch

Instructions:

1. Rinse and drain chickpeas. Chop vegetables.
2. Toss chickpeas and vegetables with lemon juice, olive oil, and cumin.
3. Garnish with fresh herbs before serving.

Nutritional Information:

- High in fibre, protein, and vitamins.

Serving Suggestions:

- Serve over a bed of greens for added freshness.
- Top with crumbled feta cheese or olives.

11. Vegetable and Lentil Stir-Fry

Ingredients:

- Mixed vegetables (bell peppers, broccoli, carrots)
- Cooked lentils
- Tamari sauce, garlic, ginger
- Brown rice or quinoa

Preparation Time: 15 minutes
Cooking Time: 20 minutes
Serving Time: Lunch

Instructions:

1. Stir-fry mixed vegetables with garlic and ginger.
2. Add cooked lentils and tamari sauce. Cook until heated through.
3. Serve over brown rice or quinoa.

Nutritional Information:

- Provides a balance of protein, fibre, and essential nutrients.

Serving Suggestions:

- Garnish with sliced green onions or sesame seeds.
- Drizzle with a homemade peanut sauce for extra flavour.

12. Spinach and Chickpea Salad with Lemon-Tahini Dressing

Ingredients:

- Baby spinach
- Canned chickpeas
- Cherry tomatoes, cucumber, red onion
- Lemon juice, tahini, garlic
- Olive oil, salt, pepper

Preparation Time: 15 minutes
Cooking Time: 0 minutes
Serving Time: Lunch

Instructions:

1. Rinse and drain chickpeas. Chop vegetables.
2. Toss spinach, chickpeas, and vegetables in a large bowl.
3. Whisk together lemon juice, tahini, garlic, olive oil, salt, and pepper for dressing.
4. Drizzle dressing over salad and toss to combine.

Nutritional Information:

- Rich in vitamins, minerals, and plant-based protein.

Serving Suggestions:

- Sprinkle with toasted pine nuts or sunflower seeds.
- Serve with a side of whole grain bread or crackers.

13. Vegetable and Lentil Curry

Ingredients:

- Mixed vegetables (cauliflower, peas, carrots)
- Cooked brown lentils
- Curry powder, coconut milk, garlic, onion
- Basmati rice or naan bread

Preparation Time: 20 minutes
Cooking Time: 25 minutes
Serving Time: Lunch

Instructions:

1. Sauté onions and garlic. Add curry powder and vegetables.
2. Stir in cooked lentils and coconut milk. Simmer until vegetables are tender.
3. Serve with basmati rice or naan bread.

Nutritional Information:

- Provides protein, fibre, and essential vitamins and minerals.

Serving Suggestions:

- Garnish with fresh cilantro and a squeeze of lime juice.
- Serve with a side of mango chutney for sweetness.

14. Sesame-Ginger Tofu Stir-Fry

Ingredients:

- Extra-firm tofu, cubed
- Mixed vegetables (bell peppers, broccoli, snap peas)
- Tamari sauce, sesame oil, ginger
- Brown rice or noodles

Preparation Time: 20 minutes
Cooking Time: 20 minutes
Serving Time: Lunch

Instructions:

1. Sauté tofu in sesame oil and ginger until golden brown.
2. Add mixed vegetables and tamari sauce. Stir-fry until vegetables are tender.
3. Serve over brown rice or noodles.

Nutritional Information:

- Rich in plant-based protein, fibre, and antioxidants.

Serving Suggestions:

- Sprinkle with toasted sesame seeds for added crunch.
- Serve with a side of kimchi or pickled vegetables.

15. Coconut-Curry Quinoa Bowl

Ingredients:

- Quinoa, cooked
- Mixed vegetables (bell peppers, snap peas, carrots)
- Curry paste, coconut milk, garlic, onion
- Fresh cilantro for garnish

Preparation Time: 15 minutes
Cooking Time: 20 minutes
Serving Time: Lunch

Instructions:

1. Sauté onions and garlic. Add curry paste and vegetables.
2. Stir in cooked quinoa and coconut milk. Simmer until vegetables are tender.
3. Garnish with fresh cilantro before serving.

Nutritional Information:

- Contains protein, fibre, and healthy fats from quinoa and coconut milk.
- Rich in vitamins and minerals from mixed vegetables.

Serving Suggestions:

- Add a squeeze of lime juice for a citrusy kick.
- Serve with a side of mango salsa for sweetness.

Ayurvedic Dinner Recipes for Endomorphs

1. Quinoa and Vegetable Stir-Fry

Ingredients:

- 1 cup quinoa
- Assorted vegetables (such as bell peppers, broccoli, carrots, and snow peas)
- 2 tablespoons olive oil
- 2 cloves garlic, minced
- 1 teaspoon grated ginger
- 2 tablespoons soy sauce
- Salt and pepper to taste

Preparation Time: 10 minutes

Cooking Time: 20 minutes

Serving Time: 30 minutes

Instructions:

1. Cook quinoa according to package instructions.
2. Heat olive oil in a large skillet over medium heat. Add minced garlic and grated ginger, sauté for 1-2 minutes.
3. Add assorted vegetables to the skillet and cook until tender-crisp.
4. Stir in cooked quinoa and soy sauce, tossing to combine.

5. Season with salt and pepper to taste.
6. Serve hot.

Nutritional Information:
- Calories: 250 per serving
- Protein: 8g
- Carbohydrates: 35g
- Fat: 9g

Serving Suggestions:
- Garnish with chopped cilantro and a squeeze of fresh lime juice.
- Serve with a side of steamed edamame beans for added protein.

2. **Lentil Soup with Spinach**

Ingredients:
- 1 cup dried lentils
- 4 cups vegetable broth
- 1 onion, diced
- 2 carrots, diced
- 2 celery stalks, diced
- 2 cloves garlic, minced
- 2 cups fresh spinach leaves
- 1 teaspoon ground cumin

- Salt and pepper to taste

Preparation Time: 10 minutes

Cooking Time: 30 minutes

Serving Time: 40 minutes

Instructions:

1. Rinse lentils under cold water and drain.
2. In a large pot, sauté diced onion, carrots, celery, and garlic until softened.
3. Add lentils and vegetable broth to the pot, bring to a boil, then reduce heat and simmer for 25-30 minutes until lentils are tender.
4. Stir in fresh spinach leaves and ground cumin, cooking until spinach wilts.
5. Season with salt and pepper to taste.
6. Serve hot.

Nutritional Information:

- Calories: 220 per serving
- Protein: 12g
- Carbohydrates: 38g
- Fat: 1g

Serving Suggestions:

- Top with a dollop of Greek yogurt and a sprinkle of chopped fresh parsley.
- Serve with a slice of whole-grain bread for a complete meal.

3. **Vegetable Curry with Brown Rice**

Ingredients:

- 1 cup brown rice
- Assorted vegetables (such as cauliflower, carrots, potatoes, and peas)
- 1 onion, diced
- 2 cloves garlic, minced
- 1 tablespoon curry powder
- 1 can (14 oz) coconut milk
- 2 tablespoons olive oil
- Salt and pepper to taste

Preparation Time: 10 minutes

Cooking Time: 40 minutes

Serving Time: 50 minutes

Instructions:

1. Cook brown rice according to package instructions.
2. In a large skillet, heat olive oil over medium heat. Add diced onion and minced garlic, sauté until softened.
3. Add assorted vegetables to the skillet and cook until slightly tender.
4. Stir in curry powder and cook for 1-2 minutes until fragrant.
5. Pour in coconut milk, stirring to combine. Simmer for 15-20 minutes until vegetables are cooked through and sauce thickens.
6. Season with salt and pepper to taste.
7. Serve hot over cooked brown rice.

Nutritional Information:

- Calories: 320 per serving
- Protein: 8g
- Carbohydrates: 40g
- Fat: 15g

Serving Suggestions:

- Sprinkle with chopped cilantro and a squeeze of fresh lemon juice.
- Serve with a side of mango chutney and naan bread for a complete Indian-inspired meal.

4. Millet and Vegetable Pilaf

Ingredients: 1 cup millet

1. Assorted vegetables (such as zucchini, bell peppers, mushrooms, and cherry tomatoes)
2. 2 tablespoons olive oil
3. 2 cloves garlic, minced
4. 1 teaspoon dried thyme
5. 4 cups vegetable broth
6. Salt and pepper to taste

Preparation Time: 10 minutes

Cooking Time: 25 minutes

Serving Time: 35 minutes

Instructions:

1. Rinse millet under cold water and drain.
2. In a large pot, heat olive oil over medium heat. Add minced garlic and sauté until fragrant.
3. Add assorted vegetables to the pot and cook until slightly tender.
4. Stir in dried thyme and rinsed millet, cooking for 1-2 minutes.
5. Pour vegetable broth into the pot, bring to a boil, then reduce heat and simmer for 15-20 minutes until millet is cooked and liquid is absorbed.
6. Season with salt and pepper to taste.

7. Serve hot.

Nutritional Information:

- Calories: 280 per serving
- Protein: 6g
- Carbohydrates: 45g
- Fat: 8g

Serving Suggestions:

- Garnish with toasted pine nuts or slivered almonds for added crunch.
- Serve with a side of steamed green beans or roasted root vegetables.

5. **Chickpea and Vegetable Tagine**

Ingredients:

- 1 can (15 oz) chickpeas, drained and rinsed
- Assorted vegetables (such as eggplant, bell peppers, carrots, and zucchini)
- 1 onion, diced
- 2 cloves garlic, minced
- 1 teaspoon ground cumin
- 1 teaspoon ground coriander
- 1 teaspoon ground cinnamon
- 1 can (14 oz) diced tomatoes
- 2 cups vegetable broth

- 2 tablespoons olive oil
- Salt and pepper to taste

Preparation Time: 15 minutes

Cooking Time: 40 minutes

Serving Time: 55 minutes

Instructions:

1. In a large skillet, heat olive oil over medium heat. Add diced onion and minced garlic, sauté until softened.
2. Add assorted vegetables to the skillet and cook until slightly tender.
3. Stir in ground cumin, ground coriander, and ground cinnamon, cooking for 1-2 minutes until fragrant.
4. Pour diced tomatoes and vegetable broth into the skillet, stirring to combine. Bring to a simmer.
5. Add drained chickpeas to the skillet, stirring to incorporate.
6. Cover and simmer for 25-30 minutes until vegetables are cooked through and flavours meld.
7. Season with salt and pepper to taste.
8. Serve hot.

Nutritional Information:

- Calories: 290 per serving
- Protein: 9g
- Carbohydrates: 45g
- Fat: 8g

Serving Suggestions:

- Serve over cooked couscous or quinoa for a complete meal.
- Garnish with chopped fresh cilantro and a dollop of Greek yogurt.

6. **Spaghetti Squash with Roasted Vegetables**

Ingredients:

- 1 spaghetti squash
- Assorted vegetables (such as cherry tomatoes, bell peppers, onions, and mushrooms)
- 2 tablespoons olive oil
- 2 cloves garlic, minced
- 1 teaspoon dried Italian herbs (such as oregano, basil, and thyme)
- Salt and pepper to taste

Preparation Time: 10 minutes

Cooking Time: 45 minutes

Serving Time: 55 minutes

Instructions:

1. Preheat oven to 400°F (200°C).
2. Cut spaghetti squash in half lengthwise and remove seeds.
3. Place spaghetti squash halves on a baking sheet, cut side down. Roast in the oven for 30-40 minutes until tender.
4. Meanwhile, prepare the roasted vegetables. Toss assorted vegetables with olive oil, minced garlic, dried Italian herbs, salt, and pepper.
5. Spread vegetables in a single layer on a separate baking sheet. Roast in the oven for 20-25 minutes until tender and lightly browned.
6. Once spaghetti squash is cooked, use a fork to scrape the flesh into strands.
7. Serve spaghetti squash topped with roasted vegetables.

Nutritional Information:

- Calories: 230 per serving
- Protein: 5g
- Carbohydrates: 30g
- Fat: 12g

Serving Suggestions:

- Sprinkle with grated Parmesan cheese or nutritional yeast for added flavour.

- Serve with a side of mixed greens dressed with balsamic vinaigrette.

7. Stuffed Bell Peppers with Quinoa and Black Beans

Ingredients:

- 4 bell peppers (any colour), halved and seeds removed
- 1 cup cooked quinoa
- 1 can (15 oz) black beans, drained and rinsed
- 1 onion, diced
- 2 cloves garlic, minced
- 1 teaspoon ground cumin
- 1 teaspoon chili powder
- 1 cup diced tomatoes
- 1 cup vegetable broth
- 2 tablespoons olive oil
- Salt and pepper to taste

Preparation Time: 20 minutes

Cooking Time: 45 minutes

Serving Time: 65 minutes

Instructions:

1. Pour vegetable broth into the skillet and add diced tomatoes. Simmer for 10-15 minutes until flavours meld and the mixture thickens.

2. Season with salt and pepper to taste.

3. While the mixture simmers, prepare the bell peppers. Place halved bell peppers in a baking dish.

4. Spoon the quinoa and black bean mixture into each bell pepper half, pressing down gently.

5. Cover the baking dish with foil and bake in the preheated oven for 25-30 minutes until the peppers are tender.

6. Serve hot.

Nutritional Information: Calories: 280 per serving

- Protein: 10g
- Carbohydrates: 45g
- Fat: 7g

Serving Suggestions:

- Top with a dollop of guacamole or sliced avocado for added creaminess.
- Serve with a side of salsa and a sprinkle of fresh cilantro.

8. **Mushroom and Asparagus Risotto**

Ingredients:

- 1 cup Arborio rice
- 8 oz mushrooms, sliced
- 1 bunch asparagus, trimmed and cut into bite-sized pieces

- 1 onion, diced
- 2 cloves garlic, minced
- 4 cups vegetable broth, kept warm
- ½ cup dry white wine
- 2 tablespoons olive oil
- ½ cup grated Parmesan cheese (optional)
- Salt and pepper to taste

Preparation Time: 15 minutes

Cooking Time: 30 minutes

Serving Time: 45 minutes

Instructions:

1. In a large pan, heat olive oil over medium heat. Add diced onion and minced garlic, sauté until softened.
2. Add sliced mushrooms and asparagus to the pan, cooking until vegetables are slightly tender.
3. Stir in Arborio rice, coating it with the oil and vegetables.
4. Pour in the white wine, stirring constantly until the liquid is mostly absorbed.
5. Begin adding warm vegetable broth, one ladle at a time, stirring frequently. Allow the liquid to be absorbed before adding more.
6. Continue this process until the rice is creamy and cooked to al dente.

7. Season with salt and pepper to taste.
8. If desired, stir in grated Parmesan cheese for added creaminess.
9. Serve hot.

Nutritional Information:
- Calories: 300 per serving
- Protein: 7g
- Carbohydrates: 55g
- Fat: 6g

Serving Suggestions:
- Garnish with chopped fresh parsley or basil for a burst of freshness.
- Serve with a side of roasted cherry tomatoes or a mixed green salad.

9. **Cauliflower and Chickpea Curry**

Ingredients:
- 1 cauliflower, cut into florets
- 1 can (15 oz) chickpeas, drained and rinsed
- 1 onion, diced
- 2 cloves garlic, minced
- 1 can (14 oz) coconut milk
- 2 tablespoons curry powder
- 2 tablespoons olive oil

- Fresh cilantro for garnish
- Salt and pepper to taste

Preparation Time: 15 minutes

Cooking Time: 40 minutes

Serving Time: 55 minutes

Instructions:

1. In a large skillet, heat olive oil over medium heat. Add diced onion and minced garlic, sauté until softened.
2. Add cauliflower florets to the skillet, cooking until slightly browned.
3. Stir in curry powder, coating the cauliflower and onions evenly.
4. Pour in coconut milk and add chickpeas, stirring to combine.
5. Cover the skillet and simmer for 25-30 minutes until cauliflower is tender.
6. Season with salt and pepper to taste.
7. Garnish with fresh cilantro before serving.

Nutritional Information:

- Calories: 260 per serving
- Protein: 8g
- Carbohydrates: 30g

- Fat: 13g

Serving Suggestions:

- Serve over basmati rice or quinoa for a complete meal.
- Drizzle with a squeeze of lime juice for added brightness.

10. **Sweet Potato and Lentil Stew**

Ingredients:

- 2 sweet potatoes, peeled and diced
- 1 cup dried green or brown lentils
- 1 onion, diced
- 2 cloves garlic, minced
- 1 can (14 oz) diced tomatoes
- 4 cups vegetable broth
- 2 tablespoons olive oil
- 1 teaspoon ground cumin
- 1 teaspoon smoked paprika
- Salt and pepper to taste

Preparation Time: 20 minutes

Cooking Time: 45 minutes

Serving Time: 65 minutes

Instructions:

1. In a large pot, heat olive oil over medium heat. Add diced onion and minced garlic, sauté until softened.
2. Add diced sweet potatoes to the pot, cooking until slightly browned.
3. Stir in ground cumin and smoked paprika, coating the vegetables evenly.
4. Pour in diced tomatoes and vegetable broth, bringing to a boil.
5. Add dried lentils to the pot, reduce heat, cover, and simmer for 30-35 minutes until lentils are tender.
6. Season with salt and pepper to taste.
7. Serve hot.

Nutritional Information:

- Calories: 290 per serving
- Protein: 12g
- Carbohydrates: 50g
- Fat: 5g

Serving Suggestions:

- Top with a dollop of Greek yogurt or coconut yogurt for added creaminess.
- Serve with a side of crusty whole-grain bread or naan.

11. Spinach and Tofu Stir-Fry

Ingredients:

- 1 block (14 oz) firm tofu, pressed and cubed
- 4 cups fresh spinach leaves
- 1 bell pepper, sliced
- 1 onion, sliced
- 2 cloves garlic, minced
- 2 tablespoons soy sauce
- 1 tablespoon sesame oil
- 1 tablespoon rice vinegar
- 1 teaspoon grated ginger
- Salt and pepper to taste

Preparation Time: 15 minutes

Cooking Time: 20 minutes

Serving Time: 35 minutes

Instructions:

1. In a large skillet, heat sesame oil over medium heat. Add minced garlic and grated ginger, sauté until fragrant.
2. Add cubed tofu to the skillet, cooking until lightly browned on all sides.
3. Stir in sliced bell pepper and onion, cooking until vegetables are tender-crisp.

4. Add fresh spinach leaves to the skillet, stirring until wilted.
5. In a small bowl, whisk together soy sauce and rice vinegar. Pour over the tofu and vegetables, tossing to combine.
6. Season with salt and pepper to taste.
7. Serve hot.

Nutritional Information:
- Calories: 230 per serving
- Protein: 15g
- Carbohydrates: 15g
- Fat: 12g

Serving Suggestions:
- Sprinkle with toasted sesame seeds for added crunch and flavour.
- Serve over cooked brown rice or quinoa for a complete meal.

12. **Broccoli and Chickpea Salad**

Ingredients:
- 2 cups cooked chickpeas
- 2 cups broccoli florets, blanched
- 1 red bell pepper, diced
- ¼ cup red onion, thinly sliced

- ¼ cup fresh parsley, chopped
- 2 tablespoons olive oil
- 1 tablespoon lemon juice
- 1 teaspoon Dijon mustard
- Salt and pepper to taste

Preparation Time: 15 minutes

Cooking Time: 5 minutes

Serving Time: 20 minutes

Instructions:

1. In a large bowl, combine cooked chickpeas, blanched broccoli florets, diced red bell pepper, sliced red onion, and chopped parsley.
2. In a small bowl, whisk together olive oil, lemon juice, Dijon mustard, salt, and pepper to make the dressing.
3. Pour the dressing over the salad ingredients, tossing to coat evenly.
4. Serve chilled or at room temperature.

Nutritional Information:

- Calories: 200 per serving
- Protein: 8g
- Carbohydrates: 25g
- Fat: 8g

Serving Suggestions:

- Add crumbled feta cheese or diced avocado for extra creaminess and flavour.
- Serve over a bed of mixed greens or alongside grilled chicken or tofu.

13. **Zucchini Noodles with Pesto**

Ingredients:

- 4 medium zucchinis, spiralized into noodles
- 1 cup cherry tomatoes, halved
- ¼ cup pine nuts, toasted
- ¼ cup grated Parmesan cheese (optional)
- 2 tablespoons olive oil
- 2 cloves garlic, minced
- 1 cup fresh basil leaves
- Salt and pepper to taste

Preparation Time: 15 minutes

Cooking Time: 5 minutes

Serving Time: 20 minutes

Instructions:

1. In a large skillet, heat olive oil over medium heat. Add minced garlic and sauté until fragrant.
2. Add zucchini noodles to the skillet, tossing until heated through but still crisp.

3. Stir in cherry tomatoes and toasted pine nuts, cooking for an additional 1-2 minutes.

4. In a food processor or blender, combine fresh basil leaves, olive oil, garlic, and Parmesan cheese (if using). Blend until smooth to make the pesto sauce.

5. Pour the pesto sauce over the zucchini noodles, tossing to coat evenly.

6. Season with salt and pepper to taste.

7. Serve hot.

Nutritional Information:

- Calories: 180 per serving
- Protein: 5g
- Carbohydrates: 10g
- Fat: 14g

Serving Suggestions:

- Garnish with additional toasted pine nuts and a sprinkle of grated Parmesan cheese.
- Serve with a side of garlic bread or grilled shrimp for added protein.

14. **Cabbage and Carrot Slaw**

Ingredients:

- ½ head green cabbage, thinly sliced
- 2 carrots, grated
- ¼ cup sliced almonds, toasted

- ¼ cup dried cranberries
- 2 tablespoons olive oil
- 2 tablespoons apple cider vinegar
- 1 teaspoon honey
- Salt and pepper to taste

Preparation Time: 15 minutes

Cooking Time: 0 minutes

Serving Time: 15 minutes

Instructions:

1. In a large bowl, combine thinly sliced green cabbage, grated carrots, toasted sliced almonds, and dried cranberries.
2. In a small bowl, whisk together olive oil, apple cider vinegar, honey, salt, and pepper to make the dressing.
3. Pour the dressing over the slaw ingredients, tossing to coat evenly.
4. Serve chilled or at room temperature.

Nutritional Information:

- Calories: 150 per serving
- Protein: 4g
- Carbohydrates: 15g
- Fat: 9g

Serving Suggestions:

- Add shredded chicken or tofu for added protein and texture.
- Serve as a side dish alongside grilled fish or roasted vegetables.

15. **Vegetable and Lentil Soup**

Ingredients:

- 1 cup dried green or brown lentils
- 4 cups vegetable broth
- 1 onion, diced
- 2 carrots, diced
- 2 celery stalks, diced
- 2 cloves garlic, minced
- 1 can (14 oz) diced tomatoes
- 2 cups chopped kale or spinach leaves
- 1 teaspoon dried thyme
- Salt and pepper to taste

Preparation Time: 15 minutes

Cooking Time: 40 minutes

Serving Time: 55 minutes

Instructions:

1. Rinse lentils under cold water and drain.
2. In a large pot, sauté diced onion, carrots, celery, and garlic until softened.
3. Add lentils and vegetable broth to the pot, bring to a boil, then reduce heat and simmer for 25-30 minutes until lentils are tender.
4. Stir in diced tomatoes, chopped kale or spinach leaves, and dried thyme, cooking until greens are wilted.
5. Season with salt and pepper to taste.
6. Serve hot.

Nutritional Information:

- Calories: 220 per serving
- Protein: 12g
- Carbohydrates: 38g
- Fat: 1g

Serving Suggestions:

- Top with a dollop of Greek yogurt or sour cream for added creaminess.
- Serve with a slice of crusty whole-grain bread or a side of quinoa for a complete meal.

Ayurvedic Dessert Recipes for Endomorphs

1. Date and Nut Balls

Ingredients:

- 1 cup dates, pitted
- 1 cup mixed nuts (almonds, cashews, walnuts)
- 1 tablespoon coconut oil
- 1 teaspoon cinnamon powder
- Shredded coconut (for coating)
  - **Preparation Time:** 15 minutes
  - **Cooking Time:** 0 minutes
  - **Serving Time:** 10 minutes

Instructions:

1. In a food processor, blend dates, mixed nuts, coconut oil, and cinnamon until a sticky dough forms.
2. Roll the mixture into small balls.
3. Roll the balls in shredded coconut.
4. Place in the refrigerator for 10 minutes to set.

Nutritional Information: (per serving)

- Calories: 120
- Fat: 8g
- Carbohydrates: 12g
- Protein: 2g

Serving Suggestions:

- Serve with a drizzle of honey and a sprinkle of cinnamon.
- Enjoy with a cup of herbal tea for a relaxing treat.

2. Coconut and Cardamom Rice Pudding

Ingredients:

- ½ cup basmati rice
- 2 cups coconut milk
- ¼ cup maple syrup or honey
- 1 teaspoon ground cardamom
- ¼ cup shredded coconut
- Sliced almonds (for garnish)
    - **Preparation Time:** 5 minutes
    - **Cooking Time:** 25 minutes
    - **Serving Time:** 30 minutes

Instructions:

1. Rinse the rice under cold water until the water runs clear.
2. In a saucepan, combine rice, coconut milk, maple syrup, and cardamom.
3. Bring to a boil, then reduce heat and simmer for 20-25 minutes, stirring occasionally, until the rice is cooked and the mixture thickens.
4. Stir in shredded coconut.

5. Remove from heat and let it cool slightly.
6. Serve garnished with sliced almonds.

Nutritional Information: (per serving)

- Calories: 250
- Fat: 14g
- Carbohydrates: 29g
- Protein: 3g

Serving Suggestions:

- Sprinkle with a pinch of ground cinnamon for extra flavour.
- Serve warm with a dollop of coconut yogurt for added creaminess.

3. Mango Lassi

Ingredients:

- 1 ripe mango, peeled and diced
- 1 cup plain yogurt or coconut yogurt
- ½ cup cold water
- 2 tablespoons honey or maple syrup
- ½ teaspoon ground cardamom
- Ice cubes (optional)
  - **Preparation Time:** 5 minutes
  - **Cooking Time:** 0 minutes
  - **Serving Time:** 5 minutes

Instructions:

1. In a blender, combine mango, yogurt, water, honey, and cardamom.
2. Blend until smooth and creamy.
3. Add ice cubes if desired and blend again until smooth.
4. Pour into glasses and serve chilled.

Nutritional Information: (per serving)

- Calories: 150
- Fat: 2g
- Carbohydrates: 32g
- Protein: 5g

Serving Suggestions:

- Garnish with a sprinkle of ground pistachios for added texture.
- Serve alongside a plate of fresh mango slices for a refreshing contrast.

4. Cardamom and Pistachio Halva

Ingredients:

- 1 cup semolina
- 1/4 cup ghee or coconut oil
- ½ cup sugar or jaggery
- 2 cups water
- ¼ cup chopped pistachios

- ½ teaspoon ground cardamom
  - **Preparation Time:** 10 minutes
  - **Cooking Time:** 20 minutes
  - **Serving Time:** 30 minutes

Instructions:

1. Heat ghee or coconut oil in a pan over medium heat.
2. Add semolina and roast until golden brown and fragrant.
3. In a separate saucepan, combine water and sugar or jaggery, and bring to a boil.
4. Gradually add the sugar syrup to the roasted semolina, stirring continuously to prevent lumps.
5. Cook until the mixture thickens and begins to pull away from the sides of the pan.
6. Stir in chopped pistachios and ground cardamom.
7. Transfer the halva to a serving dish and allow it to cool before serving.

Nutritional Information: (per serving)

- Calories: 220
- Fat: 8g
- Carbohydrates: 34g
- Protein: 4g

Serving Suggestions:

- Serve warm with a dollop of Greek yogurt for added creaminess.
- Garnish with a sprinkle of saffron threads for a touch of luxury.

5. Almond and Date Bliss Balls

Ingredients:

- 1 cup almonds, soaked and drained
- 1 cup dates, pitted
- 2 tablespoons raw cacao powder
- ¼ teaspoon vanilla extract
- Pinch of sea salt
- Desiccated coconut, for rolling
  - **Preparation Time:** 15 minutes
  - **Cooking Time:** 0 minutes
  - **Serving Time:** 15 minutes

Instructions:

1. In a food processor, blend almonds until finely ground.
2. Add dates, cacao powder, vanilla extract, and sea salt, and blend until mixture forms a sticky dough.
3. Roll mixture into small balls using your hands.
4. Roll balls in desiccated coconut until evenly coated.
5. Place in the refrigerator for 10-15 minutes to firm up.

Nutritional Information: (per serving)

- Calories: 120
- Fat: 6g
- Carbohydrates: 16g
- Protein: 3g

Serving Suggestions:

- Enjoy as a post-workout snack to replenish energy stores.
- Serve alongside a cup of herbal tea for a comforting treat.

6. Spiced Apple Compote

Ingredients:

- 4 apples, peeled, cored, and diced
- 1 tablespoon ghee or coconut oil
- 2 tablespoons maple syrup or honey
- 1 teaspoon ground cinnamon
- Pinch of ground nutmeg
  - **Preparation Time:** 10 minutes
  - **Cooking Time:** 15 minutes
  - **Serving Time:** 25 minutes

Instructions:

1. In a saucepan, melt ghee or coconut oil over medium heat.
2. Add diced apples, maple syrup, cinnamon, and nutmeg.
3. Cook, stirring occasionally, until apples are soft and caramelized, about 15 minutes.
4. Mash lightly with a fork for desired consistency.

Nutritional Information: (per serving)

- Calories: 100
- Fat: 3g
- Carbohydrates: 20g
- Protein: 1g

Serving Suggestions:

- Serve warm over Greek yogurt or coconut yogurt for added creaminess.
- Top with a sprinkle of chopped almonds for extra crunch.

7. Turmeric Golden Milk Popsicles

Ingredients:

- 2 cups coconut milk
- 1 teaspoon ground turmeric
- ½ teaspoon ground cinnamon
- ¼ teaspoon ground ginger
- 2 tablespoons honey or maple syrup

- Pinch of black pepper

Preparation Time: 5 minutes

- **Freezing Time:** 4 hours
- **Serving Time:** 4 hours 5 minutes

Instructions:

1. In a blender, combine coconut milk, turmeric, cinnamon, ginger, honey or maple syrup, and black pepper.
2. Blend until smooth and well combined.
3. Pour the mixture into popsicle molds.
4. Insert popsicle sticks and freeze for at least 4 hours, or until completely frozen.
5. To remove popsicles from molds, briefly run warm water over the outside of the molds.

Nutritional Information: (per serving)

- Calories: 150
- Fat: 12g
- Carbohydrates: 10g
- Protein: 1g

Serving Suggestions:

- Dust with a sprinkle of ground turmeric for a vibrant touch.
- Serve with a drizzle of melted dark chocolate for an indulgent twist.

8. Chia Seed Pudding with Berries

Ingredients:

- ¼ cup chia seeds
- 1 cup coconut milk or almond milk
- 1 tablespoon honey or maple syrup
- ½ teaspoon vanilla extract
- Mixed berries for topping

Preparation Time: 5 minutes

- **Chilling Time:** 2 hours
- **Serving Time:** 2 hours 5 minutes

Instructions:

1. In a bowl, whisk together chia seeds, coconut milk or almond milk, honey or maple syrup, and vanilla extract.
2. Let the mixture sit for 5 minutes, then whisk again to prevent clumping.
3. Cover and refrigerate for at least 2 hours, or until the pudding thickens.
4. Serve topped with mixed berries.

Nutritional Information: (per serving)

- Calories: 120
- Fat: 7g
- Carbohydrates: 12g
- Protein: 3g

Serving Suggestions:

- Sprinkle with a handful of toasted coconut flakes for added texture.
- Serve with a dollop of whipped coconut cream for extra creaminess.

9. Cardamom Saffron Rice Pudding

Ingredients:

- ½ cup basmati rice
- 2 cups coconut milk or almond milk
- ¼ cup honey or maple syrup
- ¼ teaspoon ground cardamom
- Pinch of saffron threads
- Chopped pistachios for garnish
  - **Preparation Time:** 5 minutes
  - **Cooking Time:** 25 minutes
  - **Serving Time:** 30 minutes

Instructions:

1. Rinse the rice under cold water until the water runs clear.
2. In a saucepan, combine rice, coconut milk or almond milk, honey or maple syrup, cardamom, and saffron threads.

3. Bring to a boil, then reduce heat and simmer for 20-25 minutes, stirring occasionally, until the rice is cooked and the mixture thickens.
4. Remove from heat and let it cool slightly.
5. Serve garnished with chopped pistachios.

Nutritional Information: (per serving)

- Calories: 200
- Fat: 8g
- Carbohydrates: 30g
- Protein: 3g

Serving Suggestions:

- Sprinkle with a pinch of ground cinnamon for extra flavour.
- Serve warm with a drizzle of honey for added sweetness.

10. Baked Apples with Cinnamon and Walnuts

Ingredients:

- 4 apples, cored
- ¼ cup chopped walnuts
- 2 tablespoons honey or maple syrup
- 1 teaspoon ground cinnamon
- ¼ teaspoon ground nutmeg
- 1 tablespoon ghee or coconut oil

- **Preparation Time:** 10 minutes
- **Cooking Time:** 25 minutes
- **Serving Time:** 35 minutes

Instructions:

1. Preheat the oven to 375°F (190°C).
2. In a bowl, combine chopped walnuts, honey or maple syrup, cinnamon, and nutmeg.
3. Stuff each cored apple with the walnut mixture.
4. Place stuffed apples in a baking dish and dot the tops with ghee or coconut oil.
5. Bake for 25-30 minutes, or until apples are tender and caramelized.

Nutritional Information: (per serving)

- Calories: 180
- Fat: 7g
- Carbohydrates: 30g
- Protein: 2g

Serving Suggestions:

- Serve warm with a scoop of vanilla ice cream or coconut yogurt.
- Garnish with a sprinkle of chopped fresh mint leaves for a burst of freshness.

CHAPTER 5

SAMPLE MEAL PLAN

Week 1:

Day 1:

- **Breakfast:** Mango Lassi
- **Lunch:** Spiced Apple Compote
- **Dinner:** Coconut and Cardamom Rice Pudding
- **Dessert:** Date and Nut Balls

Day 2:

- **Breakfast:** Turmeric Golden Milk Popsicles
- **Lunch:** Baked Apples with Cinnamon and Walnuts
- **Dinner:** Lentil Soup with Cumin and Coriander
- **Dessert:** Chia Seed Pudding with Berries

Day 3:

- **Breakfast:** Almond and Date Bliss Balls
- **Lunch:** Mixed Vegetable Stir-Fry with Ginger and Turmeric
- **Dinner:** Lentil and Vegetable Curry with Basmati Rice
- **Dessert:** Cardamom Saffron Rice Pudding

Day 4:

- **Breakfast:** Ginger and Turmeric Tea Blend
- **Lunch:** Spinach and Lentil Salad with Lemon Dressing
- **Dinner:** Vegetable Kitchari with Cumin and Coriander
- **Dessert:** Aloe Vera Juice

Day 5:

- **Breakfast:** Triphala Capsules (Herbal Supplement)
- **Lunch:** Quinoa Salad with Roasted Vegetables and Lemon-Tahini Dressing
- **Dinner:** Stuffed Bell Peppers with Quinoa and Spices
- **Dessert:** Turmeric and Boswellia Capsules (Herbal Supplement)

Day 6:

- **Breakfast:** Cinnamon and Raisin Oatmeal
- **Lunch:** Chickpea and Vegetable Curry with Basmati Rice
- **Dinner:** Roasted Sweet Potatoes with Coconut Oil and Herbs
- **Dessert:** Neem Leaf Capsules (Herbal Supplement)

Day 7:

- **Breakfast:** Ayurvedic Herbal Infusion
- **Lunch:** Lentil and Vegetable Soup with Turmeric and Ginger
- **Dinner:** Quinoa Pilaf with Mixed Vegetables and Herbs
- **Dessert:** Holy Basil Tea

Week 2:

Day 8:

- **Breakfast:** Triphala Guggulu Tablets (Herbal Supplement)
- **Lunch:** Vegetable Stir-Fry with Tofu and Tamari Sauce
- **Dinner:** Vegetable Biryani with Cucumber Raita
- **Dessert:** Licorice Root Tea

Day 9:

- **Breakfast:** Cumin and Coriander Digestive Tea
- **Lunch:** Lentil and Spinach Salad with Balsamic Vinaigrette
- **Dinner:** Baked Eggplant Parmesan with Tomato Sauce
- **Dessert:** Fennel Seed Infusion

Day 10:

- **Breakfast:** Ginger and Turmeric Smoothie with Banana and Pineapple
- **Lunch:** Quinoa and Black Bean Burrito Bowl with Avocado
- **Dinner:** Vegetable Stir-Fry with Brown Rice and Teriyaki Sauce
- **Dessert:** Guggul Extract Capsules (Herbal Supplement)

Day 11:

- **Breakfast:** Oatmeal with Cinnamon and Apple Slices
- **Lunch:** Chickpea Salad with Cucumber, Tomato, and Lemon Dressing
- **Dinner:** Vegetable Lasagna with Cashew Cheese and Marinara Sauce
- **Dessert:** Ashwagandha and Shatavari Blend (Herbal Supplement)

Day 12:

- **Breakfast:** Amla Juice
- **Lunch:** Lentil and Kale Soup with Turmeric and Garlic
- **Dinner:** Stuffed Zucchini Boats with Quinoa and Tomato Sauce
- **Dessert:** Musta Tea

Day 13:

- **Breakfast:** Mixed Berry Smoothie with Spinach and Almond Milk
- **Lunch:** Quinoa and Chickpea Salad with Lemon-Herb Dressing
- **Dinner:** Lentil Shepherd's Pie with Mashed Cauliflower
- **Dessert:** Bitter Melon Capsules (Herbal Supplement)

Day 14:

- **Breakfast:** Papaya and Lime Smoothie
- **Lunch:** Roasted Vegetable Wrap with Hummus and Sprouts
- **Dinner:** Mushroom Risotto with Arborio Rice and White Wine
- **Dessert:** Vidanga Capsules (Herbal Supplement)

Week 3:

Day 15:

- **Breakfast:** Triphala Capsules (Herbal Supplement)
- **Lunch:** Mediterranean Quinoa Salad with Olives, Tomatoes, and Feta Cheese
- **Dinner:** Roasted Vegetable and Lentil Salad with Balsamic Vinaigrette
- **Dessert:** Cumin and Coriander Digestive Tea

Day 16:

- **Breakfast:** Turmeric Golden Milk Latte
- **Lunch:** Lentil and Vegetable Curry with Basmati Rice
- **Dinner:** Spaghetti Squash with Tomato Sauce and Basil
- **Dessert:** Aloe Vera Juice

Day 17:

- **Breakfast:** Almond and Date Bliss Balls
- **Lunch:** Chickpea and Kale Salad with Lemon-Tahini Dressing
- **Dinner:** Quinoa Stuffed Bell Peppers with Black Beans and Corn
- **Dessert:** Licorice Root Tea

Day 18:

- **Breakfast:** Ginger and Turmeric Tea Blend
- **Lunch:** Mediterranean Chickpea Wrap with Hummus and Fresh Vegetables
- **Dinner:** Vegetable Stir-Fry with Tofu and Soy Sauce
- **Dessert:** Neem Leaf Capsules (Herbal Supplement)

Day 19:

- **Breakfast:** Ayurvedic Herbal Infusion
- **Lunch:** Quinoa and Black Bean Salad with Avocado and Lime Dressing

- **Dinner:** Cauliflower Fried Rice with Mixed Vegetables and Tamari Sauce
- **Dessert:** Fennel Seed Infusion

Day 20:

- **Breakfast:** Cinnamon and Raisin Oatmeal
- **Lunch:** Lentil and Vegetable Soup with Turmeric and Ginger
- **Dinner:** Zucchini Noodles with Pesto and Cherry Tomatoes
- **Dessert:** Holy Basil Tea

Day 21:

- **Breakfast:** Triphala Guggulu Tablets (Herbal Supplement)
- **Lunch:** Quinoa Salad with Roasted Vegetables and Lemon-Tahini Dressing
- **Dinner:** Vegetable Korma with Basmati Rice and Naan Bread
- **Dessert:** Guggul Extract Capsules (Herbal Supplement)

Week 4:

Day 22:

- **Breakfast:** Cumin and Coriander Digestive Tea
- **Lunch:** Lentil and Spinach Salad with Balsamic Vinaigrette
- **Dinner:** Eggplant and Chickpea Tagine with Couscous
- **Dessert:** Ashwagandha and Shatavari Blend (Herbal Supplement)

Day 23:

- **Breakfast:** Amla Juice
- **Lunch:** Quinoa and Black Bean Burrito Bowl with Avocado and Salsa
- **Dinner:** Stir-Fried Tofu with Broccoli and Teriyaki Sauce
- **Dessert:** Musta Tea

Day 24:

- **Breakfast:** Mixed Berry Smoothie with Spinach and Almond Milk
- **Lunch:** Lentil and Kale Soup with Turmeric and Garlic
- **Dinner:** Spaghetti Squash with Marinara Sauce and Meatballs
- **Dessert:** Bitter Melon Capsules (Herbal Supplement)

Day 25:

- **Breakfast:** Papaya and Lime Smoothie
- **Lunch:** Roasted Vegetable Wrap with Hummus and Sprouts
- **Dinner:** Mushroom Risotto with Arborio Rice and White Wine
- **Dessert:** Vidanga Capsules (Herbal Supplement)

Day 26:

- **Breakfast:** Triphala Capsules (Herbal Supplement)
- **Lunch:** Quinoa and Chickpea Salad with Lemon-Herb Dressing
- **Dinner:** Lentil Shepherd's Pie with Mashed Cauliflower
- **Dessert:** Bitter Melon Capsules (Herbal Supplement)

Day 27:

- **Breakfast:** Ayurvedic Herbal Infusion
- **Lunch:** Lentil and Vegetable Soup with Turmeric and Ginger
- **Dinner:** Quinoa Pilaf with Mixed Vegetables and Herbs
- **Dessert:** Holy Basil Tea

Day 28:

- **Breakfast:** Triphala Guggulu Tablets (Herbal Supplement)
- **Lunch:** Quinoa Salad with Roasted Vegetables and Lemon-Tahini Dressing
- **Dinner:** Vegetable Korma with Basmati Rice and Naan Bread
- **Dessert:** Guggul Extract Capsules (Herbal Supplement)

CHAPTER 6

HERBAL REMEDIES FOR WEIGHT MANAGEMENT

Ayurvedic Herbs for Metabolism and Digestion

1. **Triphala**: A combination of three fruits (amalaki, bibhitaki, and haritaki) known for supporting digestion and detoxification.

2. **Ginger (Zingiber officinale)**: A warming herb that aids digestion, relieves nausea, and supports healthy metabolism.

3. **Turmeric (Curcuma longa)**: Known for its anti-inflammatory properties, turmeric supports digestive health and promotes optimal metabolism.

4. **Fennel (Foeniculum vulgare)**: A carminative herb that aids digestion, relieves bloating, and supports healthy metabolism.

5. **Cumin (Cuminum cyminum)**: Aromatic seeds that aid digestion, reduce gas and bloating, and stimulate metabolism.

6. **Coriander (Coriandrum sativum)**: Supports digestion, reduces inflammation, and helps regulate metabolism.

7. **Mint (Mentha)**: Soothes the digestive tract, relieves indigestion, and supports healthy metabolism.

8. **Ajwain (Trachyspermum ammi)**: Aids digestion, relieves flatulence, and supports healthy metabolism.

9. **Asafoetida (Ferula assa-foetida)**: Known for its digestive properties, asafoetida helps reduce gas, bloating, and indigestion.

10. **Pippali (Piper longum)**: A warming herb that supports digestion, stimulates metabolism, and enhances nutrient absorption.

11. **Aloe Vera (Aloe barbadensis)**: Supports digestive health, soothes inflammation, and aids in detoxification.

12. **Licorice (Glycyrrhiza glabra)**: Soothes the digestive tract, supports healthy stomach lining, and aids in digestion.

13. **Guduchi (Tinospora cordifolia)**: Supports liver function, boosts metabolism, and aids in detoxification.

14. **Amla (Emblica officinalis)**: Rich in vitamin C, amla supports digestion, boosts immunity, and aids in detoxification.

15. **Haritaki (Terminalia chebula)**: Supports digestive health, relieves constipation, and aids in detoxification.

16. **Bhringaraj (Eclipta alba)**: Supports liver function, aids digestion, and helps detoxify the body.

17. **Punarnava (Boerhavia diffusa)**: Supports kidney function, reduces water retention, and aids in detoxification.

18. **Guggul (Commiphora mukul)**: Supports healthy cholesterol levels, aids digestion, and boosts metabolism.

19. **Bhumyamalaki (Phyllanthus niruri)**: Supports liver function, aids digestion, and helps detoxify the body.

20. **Bilva (Aegle marmelos)**: Supports digestive health, relieves constipation, and aids in detoxification.

21. **Musta (Cyperus rotundus)**: Supports digestive health, relieves bloating, and aids in detoxification.

22. **Shatavari (Asparagus racemosus)**: Supports digestive health, soothes inflammation, and aids in detoxification.

23. **Yashtimadhu (Glycyrrhiza glabra)**: Soothes the digestive tract, supports healthy stomach lining, and aids in digestion.

24. **Kutki (Picrorhiza kurroa)**: Supports liver function, aids digestion, and helps detoxify the body.

25. **Vidanga (Embelia ribes)**: Supports digestive health, aids in detoxification, and helps reduce parasites.

26. **Arjuna (Terminalia arjuna)**: Supports heart health, aids digestion, and helps detoxify the body.

27. **Kalmegh (Andrographis paniculata)**: Supports liver function, aids digestion, and helps detoxify the body.

28. **Manjistha (Rubia cordifolia)**: Supports liver function, aids digestion, and helps detoxify the body.

29. **Neem (Azadirachta indica)**: Supports digestive health, aids in detoxification, and helps reduce inflammation.

30. **Punarnava (Boerhavia diffusa)**: Supports kidney function, reduces water retention, and aids in detoxification.

Herbal Formulas for Endomorphs

1. **Triphala Capsules**: Supports digestion, aids detoxification, and promotes healthy metabolism.

2. **Ginger and Turmeric Tea Blend**: A soothing blend that aids digestion, reduces inflammation, and supports weight management.

3. **Digestive Bitters Tincture**: Stimulates digestive juices, supports liver function, and aids in the breakdown of fats.

4. **Cumin and Coriander Digestive Tea**: A traditional remedy for sluggish digestion, bloating, and gas.

5. **Metabolism Boosting Herbal Infusion**: Combines herbs like green tea, dandelion root, and cinnamon to support metabolism and weight management.

6. **Trikatu Powder**: A blend of ginger, black pepper, and long pepper that stimulates digestion, enhances metabolism, and supports weight loss.

7. **Aloe Vera Juice**: Supports digestive health, soothes inflammation, and aids in detoxification.

8. **Licorice Root Tea**: Soothes the digestive tract, supports healthy stomach lining, and aids in digestion.

9. **Fenugreek Seed Capsules**: Supports digestion, regulates blood sugar levels, and aids in weight management.

10. **Garcinia Cambogia Extract**: Helps suppress appetite, inhibits fat production, and supports weight loss efforts.

11. **Ashwagandha and Shatavari Blend**: Supports stress management, balances hormones, and promotes overall well-being for endomorphs.

12. **Neem Leaf Capsules**: Supports digestive health, aids detoxification, and helps maintain healthy blood sugar levels.

13. **Triphala Guggulu Tablets**: Combines the benefits of triphala with guggulu resin to support digestion, metabolism, and weight management.

14. **Turmeric and Boswellia Capsules**: Supports joint health, reduces inflammation, and aids in weight management for endomorphs.

15. **Cinnamon Bark Extract**: Helps regulate blood sugar levels, supports metabolism, and aids in weight management.

16. **Holy Basil Tea**: Reduces stress, supports adrenal health, and aids in weight management by balancing cortisol levels.

17. **Bitter Melon Capsules**: Supports blood sugar regulation, aids digestion, and promotes weight management.

18. **Fennel Seed Infusion**: Soothes digestive discomfort, reduces bloating, and aids in weight management.

19. **Guggul Extract Capsules**: Supports healthy cholesterol levels, aids metabolism, and promotes weight loss.

20. **Dandelion Root Capsules**: Supports liver detoxification, aids digestion, and helps maintain healthy water balance.

CONCLUSION

In conclusion, embarking on a journey toward holistic well-being through the principles of Ayurveda offers a profound opportunity for transformation. As we've explored over the past 30 days, embracing Ayurvedic practices can revolutionize not just our diets, but our entire approach to health and vitality.

For many of us, the journey to better health can feel overwhelming and daunting. We understand the struggles and challenges that come with striving to find balance in a world filled with temptations and distractions. The path to wellness is rarely linear, and setbacks are a natural part of the process. But it's important to remember that every step forward, no matter how small, brings us closer to our goals.

Through the diverse array of Ayurvedic breakfasts, lunches, dinners, and desserts, we've discovered the power of nourishing our bodies with whole, natural foods that support digestion, metabolism, and overall vitality. From the comforting warmth of turmeric golden milk to the refreshing simplicity of a green smoothie, each meal has been carefully crafted to delight the senses and promote optimal well-being.

But beyond the recipes themselves, the essence of Ayurveda lies in the cultivation of mindfulness and self-awareness. It's about listening to our bodies, honoring their innate wisdom, and making conscious choices that align with our unique constitutions and needs. It's about finding balance in all aspects of our lives – not just on our plates, but in our relationships, our work, and our daily routines.

As we reflect on the past month, let us celebrate the progress we've made and the lessons we've learned. Let us acknowledge the moments of struggle and resistance, knowing that they too have played a vital role in our growth and evolution. And let us approach each new day with a sense of curiosity and openness, embracing the journey with courage and resilience.

Remember, transformation is not a destination but a continuous process – a journey of self-discovery and self-love. As we continue on this path, let us draw inspiration from the words of Rumi, who reminds us that "the wound is the place where the light enters you." In our vulnerabilities and imperfections, we find the seeds of our greatest strength and resilience. Let us embrace them wholeheartedly and allow them to illuminate the path toward a life of vibrant health, joy, and fulfillment.

May we carry the wisdom of Ayurveda in our hearts as we navigate the complexities of modern living, trusting in its timeless principles to guide us toward a life of balance, harmony, and well-being. And may we always remember that the power to transform lies within each of us – one mindful choice, one nourishing meal, and one day at a time.

www.ingramcontent.com/pod-product-compliance
Lightning Source LLC
Chambersburg PA
CBHW071212240526
45470CB00018B/1804